LAST WEEK
I WANTED
TO DIE

EVANGELIST ANGIE BEE

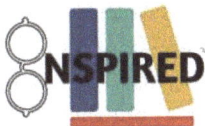

NSPIRED

Reading for the Whole Person

INSPIRED published by
Ladero Press LLC

229 Kettering Road
Deltona, Florida 32725

First Ladero Press Printing, December 2020

Last Week...I Wanted to Die

Copyright © 2020 by Angela Neal

All rights reserved.

ISBN: 978-1-946981-29-5 Paperback / 978-1-946981-30-1 Mobi /
978-1-946981-53-0 EPub

Printed in the United States of America

Set in EB Garamond

Cover Designed by LaShalonda Robinson

Library of Congress information available upon request. www.laderopress.com

DEDICATION

This book is dedicated to the memory of my mother,

Sandra Henderson Bennett

"May you never endure another cloudy day"

TABLE OF CONTENTS

Preface 7

Acknowledgements...9

Introduction Who Am I? 13

Chapter 1: It Has Begun...17

Chapter 2: Solid As A Rock 19

Chapter 3: The Frantic Styling Of Miss Lucy.......................22

Chapter 4: What Happened Last Week? 24

Chapter 5: Startling Statistics 33

Chapter 6: Trusting God In Times Of Trouble 37

Chapter 7: My Blessing And My Curse................................49

Contact The Author...58

PREFACE

— ∿ —

AUGUST 19, 2019

As I prepare for the second published edition of this, my first book, I cannot help but give God praise. I see how far I have come in just these few short years, by leaning upon the Lord. My territory has enlarged, I am safe from harm, I have a steady foundation of mental health management and I am blessed with health and love.

Thank You, Jesus!

Read this book, share this story with others and realize that there IS a light at the end of this dark tunnel when you hold firm to God's unchanging and loving hand.

BEE Blessed,
Angie BEE

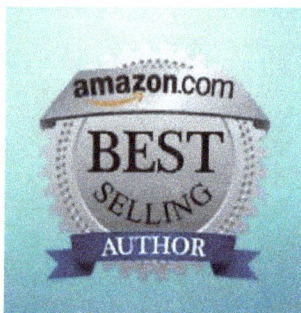

Contributing Author to:

Daily Dose of Direction for Women in Business and
Daily Dose of Declaration by Melanie Bonita

ACKNOWLEDGEMENTS

I give all honor to my Lord and CERTAIN Savior, Jesus Christ.

Jasmine, thank you for saving my life; and thank you for remaining IN my life. I love you.

I SO appreciate my daughters, Angelyn and Jasmine. It is so unfair that you had to grow up with an ill mother, but I pray that all we went through will strengthen you both as you grow older. I love you both!

Thank you to my sisters:

Sonya, you were always there when I needed someone to talk to, and you still are...you are my mini-hero!

Tanya, you will never know how good it was to come home every time you sent for me. You helped to save me. Now, please pass the sweet potatoes!

Daddy – I love you. I really, really do (tear rolls down my face). I just can't say enough about how much I love you.

Gram Gram – You opened my eyes so much. I was not alone. You knew what I was going through, but you would not let me go. I want to be a strong woman just like you. Can we go to Buddy's Pizza now?

Grandmama – If nobody else knows how to pray for me, I know that you do. If nobody knows how to pick up a bible, you do. I know that I will be okay because I have you in my life.

To my ministry families at The Lighthouse Citadel of Truth, Reconciliation Christian Center, and the Glorious Church of Christ (Orlando, Florida); Hartford Memorial Baptist Church (Detroit); and Beth Eden Missionary Baptist Church (Detroit). Each of you imparted something special in me that I still have today.

Oh, My God... Thank you. I am grateful for each of you.

To Suzie, Felecia, Bridget, Dawn, Cora Miles-Jefferson, the members of the One Accord Deejay Alliance, members of The Higher Ground International Record Pool, and to the Jericho Broadcast Network and others that knew of me and prayed for me. Thank you to each of you.

My children are thankful that you prayed for their mother; and the small child in me still feels unworthy of your intercession. I appreciate each of you.

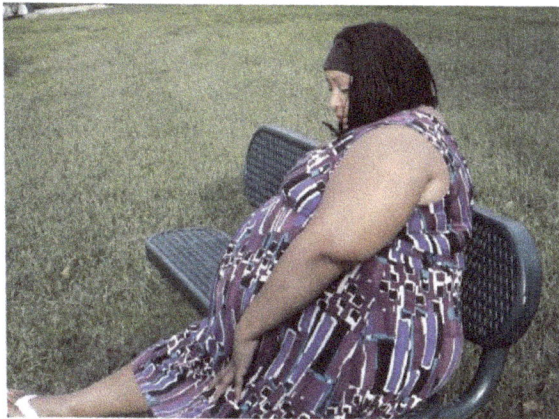

Summer of 2010
Angela at her heaviest weight of 360 pounds

During the writing of this book, Angela experienced:

Type II Diabetes
High Blood Pressure
Sleep Apnea
Peripheral Artery Disease (P.A.D.)
Generalized Anxiety Disorder
Major Depressive Disorder

INTRODUCTION
WHO AM I?

━━━━━━━━━━━ ∾ ━━━━━━━━━━━

I was born Angela Yvette Bennett on May 8th to Al James and Sandra Luvenia Bennett. My mother tells me that I was born at 9 pounds and 15 ounces, the second largest baby every born at Northwest Grace Hospital.

Growing up in Detroit, my life was filled with wonderful gifts, talents, love and family. Younger sisters made me feel responsible and a bevy of grandparents and even great grandmothers made me feel like I belonged.

During my 20s I married, had children, traveled and divorced. I started businesses and grew in understanding. In my thirties I remarried, returned to college and learned how to hear the voice of God as I tried to learn more about my spirituality.

Someone once said to me "Your life sounds like it was so perfect. It's a given that dark days should hit". Major Depressive Disorder hit me with a vengeance and not only separated me from my family, but separated me from Our God in a way like I had never experienced. After three suicide attempts, two hospitalizations and one major life re-dedication I am on the road to my healing. 3-2-1-GO! This book is the beginning of my new life. A life full of revelation. A life full of ministry. This book takes you to where I was during that time. This book lets you peek into my life.

I would be honored to come and speak to your congregation, women's group or youth group. The message of depression and healing NEEDS to be taught in our churches. I know that this message is not your usual "Love the Lord, and He will set you free!" message... but I do know that if God can speak to a man through a donkey, then He can certainly use me to speak to you.

Share this book with others. Together we may save a life and a soul.

BEE Blessed,
Angie BEE

LAST WEEK
I WANTED
TO DIE

CHAPTER 1
IT HAS BEGUN

~

"Mommy, what did you do? What did you do?"

Vanessa was shaking me. Her hands were on my shoulders and it seemed like her frantic voice was full on in my face, yelling at me! I was asleep! What was she talking about? What was she asking me? I'm asleep! I didn't do anything?!

Then, I began to hear voices all around me--almost as if everyone were standing around me.

I began to hear voices next. My eldest daughter Mallory, my best friend FeFe, and my husband Leon, all seemed to be talking to each other in loud, frantic voices. It seemed like everyone was shouting at me! What's up with my family? Can't they see that I'm trying to sleep? I am so tired; all I want to do is sleep. *Ahhh!* That breeze feels really nice on my face. Is my bedroom window open? That doesn't feel like a breeze from the ceiling fan; it feels like someone's blowing a gentle breeze across my face and shoulders...a nice, warm, loving breeze. *God. Is that you?*

"*Nine-One-One? Yes. My name is FeFe. My friend just tried to kill herself. No. Yes. Yes. No. We are all here with her. We are outside. Her name is Angela. She looks like she is awake; her eyes are open, but she will not answer us. She's not all there.*

Her husband found three or four empty medicine bottles in the bathroom. Her daughters are here with me. Yes, we are all here with her. We are talking to her, trying to keep her awake."

Who tried to kill themselves? Who was she talking about? Daughters? Empty medicine bottles? What's going on? Let me get up from this bed and go see what FeFe is talking about. Let me get up and see what's going on. *Get up?* I AM up... I'm standing... *Outside?*

CHAPTER 2
SOLID AS A ROCK

~

When I was with FeFe, I felt like I could do ANYTHING! She drove that shyness right out of me. I talked to guys, I stayed up late, I went on dates...we have road trip stories to tell that would make a person shiver, and we both buried our moms within months of each other. She has a husband who adores her and a big brother in the military. FeFe has been my best friend since college. MAN! The stories we could tell!

She was now in town for a visit, and she was the last person I remember talking to before I went to bed. She and my daughters were visiting a friend, but I was stressed and tired.

I remember arguing with my husband, and it seemed like he was getting louder and louder. I had an awful headache, and I was SO tired. My husband called our pastor, and while he spoke with him on the phone, he paced back and forth in the living room. Now, he wanted to pass the phone to me so Pastor could tell me something. I was too tired to keep my eyes open, much less hold a conversation with Pastor. With this recent bought of insomnia, all I could think of was sleep. I was sitting at the computer when Leon handed me the phone.

"Hello, Pastor?"

"Sister Angie, I am so disappointed in you. Why would you allow the devil to come into your home like this?"

What is he talking about? What did I do wrong, now? It seemed like Pastor's voice just trailed off into nothingness. Leon was still cussing and pacing the floor. Who was this on the phone? I need some sleep.

Let me call FeFe. She is my solid rock right now. Whatever Leon is complaining about can wait until morning. Pastor and I can talk during our next counseling session. FeFe is only in town for a couple of days, so let me reach out to her.

Hello, Mommy!

Vanessa always sounds so happy when I call her. You can hear the smile on her face when she answers the phone.

Hi, Baby. Let me speak to your Auntie.

FeFe was a close as family could be; so, she was always referred to as Auntie.

Hello?

Hey girl, I am headed to bed. Leon is trippin' and I have a horrible headache. I just need some sleep. I hurt all over. Are you and the girls having a good time?

Oh, yeah! We are...

That was strange. FeFe's voice just seemed to trail off in the distance somewhere... all I hear is Leon on the phone with Pastor... all I feel is pain... all I want to do is sleep.

"FeFe, listen to me. Take care of my girls for me. Take care of my girls. Okay?" I hung up the phone, and headed to the bathroom.

CHAPTER 3
THE FRANTIC
STYLING OF MISS LUCY

⟿

"Here, Angie. Lucy is on the phone."

Leon was handing me the phone. Couldn't he see that I'm asleep? What could be so important that Lucy has to have Leon to wake me up, now?

"Hello, Lucy," I said with little enthusiasm.

Lucy could be a drama queen when she wanted to be, but I loved her and wanted to be a good friend to her. Everything was a huge production with her. The dog pooping on the carpet, the next-door neighbors, and the giant spider on her ceiling; she was the queen of drama, and I catered to her. She always referred to me as her best friend, and I never corrected her. I figured that if I was the best that she has as a friend, then she really did need someone in her life.

"Hello, Lucy." I sighed heavily, but managed to get a smile on my face through the phone.

"What in the hell are you doing? What did you take? Don't you know they are going to pump your stomach? Why would you..." Her voice trailed off and sounded like background noise.

What was she talking about? I'm going back to sleep. Whatever she is fussing about will be there in the morning. It seems like EVERYBODY is upset with me about something lately. *Everybody!* I am so sleepy.

CHAPTER 4
WHAT HAPPENED LAST WEEK?

I was now an inpatient at the mental health hospital in Orlando. This one was a bit different than the one in Kissimmee. This one seemed a bit older, but the process was still the same. You stay here for at least three days, and then you are discharged. You participate in group counseling, and one-on-one counseling with a therapist, and you try to wrap your mind around what has happened to you. Now, the therapist was asking me one simple question that I could not answer...

"What happened last week?"

"What pushed you over the edge? Why are you here?"

Last week, I tried to kill myself. It was a simple act I swallowed a bottle of sleeping pills just as easily as I swallowed the glass of water to wash them down.

Why did I do it? Some would say that the stresses of life were too great for me to handle, and this was my way of no longer having to deal with issues. Some would say that I wasn't "prayed up" enough; that I wasn't "fasting" enough or that I wasn't seeking God. Others would say that years of struggling with the chemical imbalances in my brain that resulted in Major Depressive Disorder were returning with a vengeance, and that I should have reached out to "someone" for help.

All that I know is that everyone around me was disappointed with me in one way or another. My kids were tired of my irritability; my husband was frustrated because I couldn't find a job; my parents were tired of helping me financially (I mean, I DID have a husband!); and my pastor's heart was breaking because I was allowing *the devil* to get a hold of me and my family; and...my Lord and Savior must have decided that I was no longer worthy of His guidance because His voice had recently become quiet to me.

Major Depressive Disorder is a disease, just like cancer and diabetes where something in your body is not working properly and the result could be death.

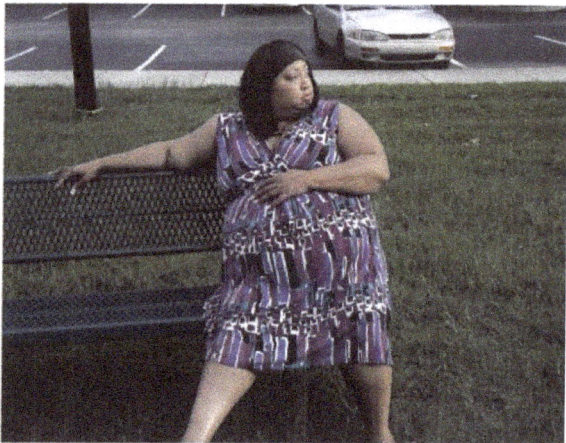

Angie's daughter Jasmine took this picture
after encouraging her to go outside

State regulations in Florida require that when an individual is suicidal, he/she must be detained in the mental health hospital for no less than 72 hours until that person is deemed "stable" and no longer a threat to him/herself.

As I was being "processed" for my admission, an angel came to me. I don't remember her name, but I remember her words, her prayers, and that warm hug she risked her job for in order to give to me...a hug from God through the arms of a State employee.

Recovery will be a long, yet pleasant road - one that I have unfortunately traveled before, but this time an angel left me with the following scriptures that I will now share with you.

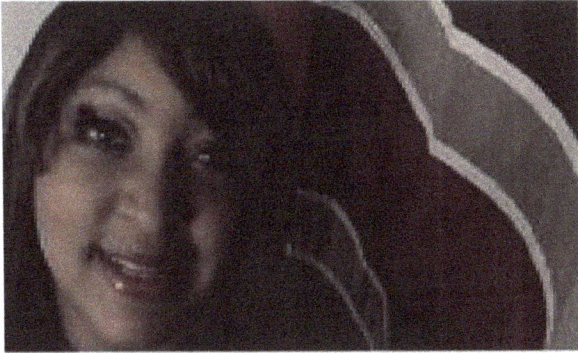

A picture of me, taken by my daughter - 2008 When you are sad, read John, Chapter 14, verses 1-4:

Don't let your hearts be troubled. Trust in God, and trust also in me. 2 There is more than enough room in my Father's home.[a] If this were not so, would I have told you that I am going to prepare a place for you? [b] 3 When everything is ready, I will come and get you, so that you will always be with me where I am. 4 And you know the way to where I am going.

The scripture also reads,

13 You can ask for anything in my name, and I will do it, so that the Son can bring glory to the Father. 14 Yes, ask me for anything in my name, and I will do it!

Finally, in verse 27: **I am leaving you with a gift— peace of mind and heart. And the peace I give is a gift the world cannot give. So don't be troubled or afraid.**

When you feel as if God is far from you, read Psalm 149.

When you are alone and scared, read Psalm 23, particularly, verse 4:

Even when I walk through the darkest valley, I will not be afraid, for you are close beside me. Your rod and your staff protect and comfort me.

When you feel like an outcast, read Romans 8:31-39:

If God is for us, who can ever be against us? 32 Since he did not spare even his own Son but gave him up for us all, won't he also give us everything else? Can anything ever separate us from Christ's love? Does it mean he no longer loves us if we have trouble or calamity, or are persecuted, or hungry, or destitute, or in danger, or threatened with death? No, despite

all these things, overwhelming victory is ours through Christ, who loved us. And I am convinced that nothing can ever separate us from God's love. Neither death nor life, neither angels nor demons,[b] neither our fears for today nor our worries about tomorrow—not even the powers of hell can separate us from

God's love. 39 No power in the sky above or in the earth below— indeed, nothing in all creation will ever be able to separate us from the love of God that is revealed in Christ Jesus our Lord.

"It is not about our situation – Give God your all – Give God your ashes, and He will turn it into beauty. The world will give you bashes for ashes, but God will give you love and acceptance" – Man with no limbs

LifeWithoutLimbs.org, as seen on The Good Life TV 45 ——The Good Life *"No matter where I am – God's arms are never too short to reach me".*

When your bank account is empty, read Psalms 37, verses 1 through 40.

Trust in the Lord and do good. Then, you will live safely in the land and prosper.

Take delight in the Lord, and he will give you your heart's desires. Commit everything you do to the Lord. Trust him, and he will help you. Psalm 37:3-5

Be still in the presence of the Lord, and wait patiently for him to act. Psalm 37:7

It is better to be godly and have little than to be evil and rich. For the strength of the wicked will be shattered, but the Lord takes care of the godly. Psalm 37:16

Day by day the Lord takes care of the innocent, and they will receive an inheritance that lasts forever. They will not be disgraced in hard times; even in famine they will have more than enough. Psalm 37:18-19

The wicked borrow and never repay, but the godly are generous givers. Psalm 37:21

Those the Lord blesses will possess the land, but those he curses will die. Psalm 37:22

When you are losing hope, read Psalm 126:5-6:

5 Those who plant in tears will harvest with shouts of joy. 6 They weep as they go to plant their seed, but they sing as they return with the harvest.

The Lord rescues the godly; he is their fortress in times of trouble. The Lord helps them, rescuing them from the wicked. He saves them, and they find shelter in him. Psalm 37:39-40

When someone is screaming at you, or if you are losing your temper, read Psalm 37, verses 8 and 9:

Stop being angry! Turn from your rage! Do not lose your temper— it only leads to harm. For the wicked will be destroyed, but those who trust in the Lord will possess the land.

When you are depressed, read Psalm 27:10-14:

Even if my father and mother abandon me, the Lord will hold me close. Teach me how to live, O Lord. Lead me along the right path, **for my enemies are waiting for me. Wait patiently for the Lord. Be brave and courageous. Yes, wait patiently for the Lord.**

Psalm 37, verse 24:

Though they stumble, they will never fall, for the Lord holds them by the hand.

There were other scriptures that were listed on this piece of paper that she slipped into my hand, but these are the ones that addressed the feelings I experienced for weeks prior to my hospitalization. It may have been just a simple sheet of paper with words on it, but to me it was like a love letter from My Father above, and it can be that way for you, too!

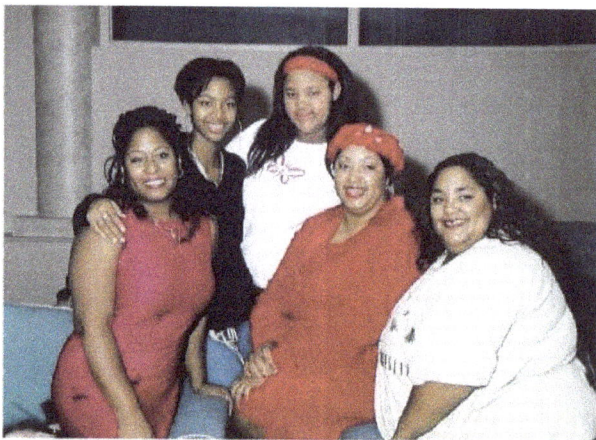

I love this picture of my daughters, sisters and me.

Clockwise: Jasmine (daughter), me, Sonya (sister), Tanya (sister) and Angelyn (daughter)

CHAPTER 5
STARTLING STATISTICS

⟿

PSAs debut at Howard University and Colleges and Universities Nationwide as part of First Annual HBCU National Mental Health Awareness Day

Washington, D.C., February 23, 2010

Mental health conditions account for more than 15 percent of the burden of disease in established market economies-more than the disease burden caused by all cancers. *NIMH*

Mental illnesses, including depression, anxiety, bipolar disorder and schizophrenia, are widespread in the U.S. and often misunderstood. According to SAMHSA, in 2008 there were an estimated 9.8 million adults aged 18 or older living with serious mental illness. Among adults, the prevalence of serious mental illness is highest in the age group of 18 to 25, yet this age group is also the least likely to receive services or counseling. In 2008, 6.0 percent of African-Americans ages 18-25 had serious mental illness in the past year. Overall, only 58.7 percent of Americans with serious mental illness received care within the past 12 months and the percentage of African-Americans receiving services is only 44.8 percent.

Terrie M. Williams, MSW, co-founder of The Stay Strong Foundation, "Every day so many of us wear the "mask" of wellness that hides our pain from the world. Now is the time to identify and name our pain—minus the myths and the stigmas—and seek the help so many of us need."

"In general, mental health problems are difficult to talk about," said Rob Baiocco, EVP/Executive Creative Director of Grey New York. "But the second someone opens up and tells their specific personal story you instantly realize what they are dealing with. It's such an immediate, intuitive and emotional understanding and from that, comes the healing."

If you know someone who is depressed or has faced suicide, these are some things that you should NOT say to them:

"Why didn't you call me?

"Are you praying? Are you fasting?"

"Everyone has problems. Why can't you face yours?"

"It couldn't have been THAT bad?"

"Are you going though Change of Life?"

"Just eat chocolate and bananas."

"You've got kids! Didn't you think of them?"

"You need to stay in that hospital until you get better because we don't want you to do this again!"

"Mommy, why did you do this? Don't you know that I need you?"

The best thing that you can do for a person that is depressed is to go and see them--spend time with them. Let them cry on your shoulder. Help them cook their meals, and remind them to shower and take care of themselves. BE WITH THEM! Don't dismiss them. Don't dismiss their feelings! Don't tell them, "You shouldn't feel like that!" They don't want to be in pain any more than you want to hurt from a cut, a broken bone, or a burn.

Don't get angry with them because they took you through this stressful time. Mostly, they did this to try and release you from the stress of having to deal with them! All I wanted to do was to make things easier for everyone else in my life by removing my problems from their lives. Don't just call them every now and then to see if they will answer the phone. Most times, they won't answer.

Suicide is the beginning of more Hell than you know what to do with – stated a renowned pastor.

If a believer knows that suicide leads to damnation, why would they even consider it?

What happens when the pain of living and hurting others becomes greater than what we know of damnation...

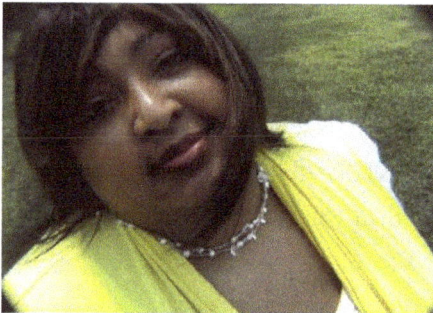

Summer of 2010

CHAPTER 6
TRUSTING GOD IN TIMES OF TROUBLE

At times, it seems like we wait to hear an audible voice from God. We wait for this voice to give us instruction or encouragement. What we fail to realize is that if God can speak to a man through a donkey, he can certainly speak to you through the TV screen.

During my healing process, I left on my TV.

The following excerpts were delivered to me through the TV preachers that I watched--words that came to me in a loud and clear voice from my Lord and Savior Jesus Christ. I acknowledge each of these ministry leaders, and I thank them for speaking into my life when I needed it most.

River of Life Christian Church, Orlando – ROLCC.tv

The Senior Pastor once said, *"Your music has a made-up mind! Make a resolve to stay healthy, to stay happy, and to stay stress free! It is ok to say NO! It is ok to do something for yourself without feeling guilty! To trust God in times of trouble – stand strong"*

Hebrews 10-35 says: **So do not throw away this confident trust in the Lord. Remember the great reward it brings you! Patient endurance is what you need now, so that you will continue to do God's will. Then you will receive all that he has promised.**

Sometimes in life you must simply trust in the Lord. Don't be weary when you are doing good – Keep the Faith! This is called the Faith Fight!! Look at the Faith Fight that Job endured!

Know that your destiny is in God's hands.

Jeremiah 29:11 tells us, **"For I know the plans I have for you,"** says the Lord. **"They are plans for good and not for disaster, to give you a future and a hope."**

The devil tested Eve's mind FIRST! Eve received her information second-hand...from Adam. Don't be fooled or confused! Get your information FIRST HAND...from God! This way, your mind can't be so easily tested!

Two other pastors stated during a Broadcast, that we should trust in the instruments provided to you! When flying an airplane, you may become upside down. Trust in what the instrument panel is telling you so that you can reach your destination – so that you can reach your destiny! Trust in the word of God when darkness is all around you! The Word of God is your light! If all you can do is pick up these 66 books and read them...if you can't see the words on the page, pick up the remote and KEEP THE TV on a Christian channel!!

If you are online, keep the gospels streaming through your speakers!!! Keep the Word around you, like the air...the Word will seep through the fog and will keep you through the darkness.

Another pastor asked the question: *"How do I let God's Word abide in me? The more I let the Word dwell in me, the better I am!"* The healthier I become! Let the healing begin in your life! Let prosperity come in and heal your *poverty!* Colossians 3:16 says *"Let the message about Christ, in all its richness, fill your lives. Teach and counsel each other with all the wisdom he gives. Sing psalms and hymns and spiritual songs to God with thankful hearts."* He further stated that God's truth shall set us free of darkness! Free of poverty! Free of sickness and despair! Speak Life. He went on to say that you should speak abundance over your life! God supplies my needs!! I speak daily – *I am strong, I am prosperous, I do not have depressions!* I will receive a blessing because of my faith! Now, my mission is to go tell people how God has blessed me! I have to share the Good News to people around the world!

I take communion over my pain and illness now, and I see Jesus bearing my pain.

When is it ok to be sad?

Ecclesiastes 7:3 reads, **"Sorrow is better than laughter: for by the sadness of the countenance the heart is made better."**

I am better because of my years of sadness. I am STRONGER because of my sadness, and I am healthier because of my sadness...and because of the grace of GOD!

A Pastor from Singapore said, *"Stress is the first thing that Jesus bore for us – the stress of knowing that His time on this Earth was coming to an end."*

He also teaches that panic attacks affect your stomach and intestines. *LOOK AT ME! Whatever you feel, affects your stomach. Now, 360 pounds later...I can't hold all that I internalized... I need medical help just to be able to stand.*

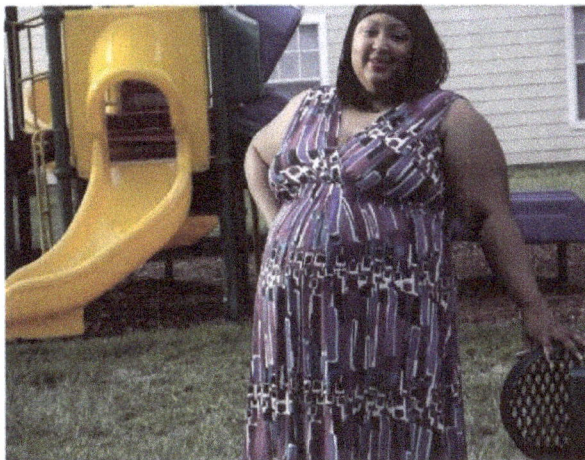

Don't be like me! Learn from me! Help someone else...you may be the only God that this person has... don't regret not doing all that you can. They need you – we need you – We love you!

If you know someone that is going through a depressive period - Pray with them and for them and bring them this book so they can see that someone else has been where they are...and that someone, was me.

The National Mental Health Information Center website says: Like adults, children and adolescents can have mental health disorders that interfere with the way they think, feel, and act. When untreated, mental health disorders can lead to *school failure, family conflicts, drug abuse, violence,* and even *suicide.* Untreated mental health disorders can be very costly to families, communities, and the health care system.

Women and Depression Fast Facts
(Source Unknown)

- One in four women will experience severe depression at some point in life.

- Depression affects twice as many women as men, regardless of racial and ethnic background or income.

- Depression is the number one cause of disability in women.

- In general, married women experience more depression than single women do, and depression is common among young mothers who stay at home full-time with small children.

- Women who are victims of sexual and physical abuse are at much greater risk for depression.

- At least 90 percent of all cases of eating disorders occur in women, and there is a strong relationship between eating disorders and depression.

- Depression can put women at risk for suicide. While more men than women die from suicide, women attempt suicide about twice as often as men do.

- Only about one-fifth of all women who suffer from depression seek treatment.

- Depression can - and should - be treated.

CENTRAL FLORIDA RESOURCES

Orlando
Devereux Florida
5850 T G Lee Blvd Ste 400
Orlando, FL 32822-4409
Phone: (407) 362-9210
Service Setting: Administrative Only

Devereux Orange Counseling Ctr/
Therapeutic Foster Care
1010 Executive Center Dr Ste100
Orlando, FL 32803
Phone: (321) 281-3840
Service Setting: Outpatient Care

Devereux Residential Treatment Center
6147 Christian Way
Orlando, FL 32808-1435
Phone: (407) 296-5300
Service Setting: Residential Care

Florida Hospital
Attn: Center for Behavioral Health
601 E Rollins St
Orlando, FL 32803-1489

Phone: (407) 303-8053

Service Setting: Inpatient and Outpatient Care

Florida Hospital Center for Behavioral H

601 E Rollins Street Box #48

Orlando, FL 32803-1248

Phone: (407) 303-8076

Service Setting: General MH ServiceLakeside

Behavioral Healthcare

Central Plaza

434 W Kennedy Blvd

Orlando, FL 32810-6228

Phone: (407) 875-3700

Service Setting: Inpatient and Outpatient Care

Lakeside Behavioral Healthcare

Princeton Plaza

1800 Mercy Dr

Orlando, FL 32808-5646

Phone: (407) 875-3700

Service Setting: Inpatient, Residential, and Outpatient
Care

Lakeside Behavioral Healthcare
Residential Plaza
4524 Thistledown Dr
Orlando, FL 32804-1244
Phone: (407) 291-6335
Service Setting: Residential Care

Orange County Youth and Family
Services Division
1718 E Michigan St
Orlando, FL 32806
Phone: (407) 836-7645
Service Setting: General MH Service

Orlando Regional South Seminole Hospital
555 W State Rd
Orlando, FL 32750-8014
Phone: (407) 767-5800

Orlando
VAMC Mental Health (116A)
5201 Raymond St
Orlando, FL 32803-8208
Phone: (407) 629-1599
Service Setting: Residential and Outpatient Care

Renaissance Healthcare Group, LLC
Pasadena Villa
119 Pasadena Pl
Orlando, FL 32803-3825
Phone: (407) 246-0887
Service Setting: Residential Care

The Devereux Foundation
Devereux Florida Treatment Network
5850 TG Lee Blvd Ste 400
Orlando, FL 32822
Phone: (800) 338-3738
Service Setting: General MH Service

University Behavioral Center
2500 Discovery Dr
Orlando, FL 32826-3711
Phone: (407) 281-7000
Service Setting: Residential and Outpatient Care

CHAPTER 7
MY BLESSING
AND MY CURSE

Anytime a person says to me:

"I have good news and bad news. Which do you want first?"

I always respond that I want the bad news first, so I can end on a positive note (LOL!).

The bad news about writing this book, sharing my testimony through speaking engagements and promoting this book on social media is that I have become a "suicide expert." Anytime a celebrity commits suicide, people on social media begin to message me. "Why", "How" "What the - -"

Anytime a social media friend loses a loved one to suicide, they contact me for prayer and comfort. I always let them know that the TRUE comforter is Jesus, and He is the truth and the way to salvation and ultimate joy. I always let them know that I am not a licensed counselor, so I cannot give advice... I can only share my story with them and pray that testimony leads them to peace and understanding.

I have heard comments over the years from people (mainly men) that have led me to lean closer to God. Some people have said to me:

"All you need is a good man in your life, and you won't be depressed anymore."

"You are such a beautiful woman! If you were with me, I would treat you like a Queen!"

"You don't need medication! You shouldn't be on disability! You can get a job and not be lazy. Ain't nothing wrong with you!"

As the years of my life thankfully continue, I have also heard comments from parents trying to raise their children. Women attending our Moms-n-Ministry workshop will cry out to God as they realize their child may be showing symptoms of mental illness. We always pray with them and for them, and we refer them to medical and psychiatric professionals.

Unfortunately, during my years in ministry, I have also heard from men--in reference to their children and the possibility of mental illness. Most of these comments have come from African American men, yet not all of them. When I hear the following statements, I cringe and ask God to give them wisdom as it relates to their children.

"Ain't nothing wrong with MY seed!"

"Ain't nobody in MY family crazy!"

"That boy/girl just want some attention."

"Ain't nothing wrong with them!"

"I don't claim that!"

Now, I want you to fast forward to January 2013. I had peace in my mind, in my body, and in my soul. I found it. I had it. I embraced it and even flaunted it; always giving God the praise. I served the Lord with gladness and anything He directed me to do or say, I did and said. Our evangelism troupe was growing and saving souls for Christ, and we had just completed a successful outreach concert in Daytona Beach, Florida. It took place at a church that allowed us to collect canned goods for their food pantry, AND they blessed us with hotel rooms! I enjoyed visiting Daytona Beach in November of 2012 - - and I never would have imagined what the Lord had planned for me just a few months later.

The TOUR was introducing our first testimonial workshop entitled "The Moms-n-Ministry". It debuted on January 25, 2013 – exactly 17 years after the devil FIRST tried to end my life in a head-on collision. As the attendees arrived to the workshop, I felt the Spirit of the Lord come upon me. I felt love, joy, peace and comfort; I led the workshop while knowing that the devil did NOT take my life back then, and he wouldn't take my life that day!

"Get behind me, Satan! You are a stumbling block to me; you do not have in mind the concerns of God, but merely human concerns." NIV

Jesus may have spoken those words to Peter in the book of Matthew 16:23, but I was claiming those words for myself to fight mental illness and to serve the Lord with my life!

I had a new Pastor and he proclaimed that I had a calling on my life; he called me a "Prophetess of the Lord." My youngest daughter had graduated high school, and was working and attending college about a two-hour drive from the new apartment that the Lord had blessed me to move in to. The car was running fine, my family in Michigan was all fine, I was happy and growing closer to the Lord each day... and then Bartee came along.

ON our first date I told him two things that I just KNEW would result in him leaving. You see, I was doing fine without a man in my life, and I didn't want to travel the emotional roller coaster of dating, falling in love, and getting hurt, so I thought I could tell him these things, and that would be it! I was NEVER going to submit to another man, especially a Black man; they leave you, disease you, and crush you. I was even angry at God (for a hot minute). I remember standing in my kitchen and saying these words out loud "God, what am I supposed to do with HIM?!" These feelings that were growing inside of me would not stop, and I wanted "he and I" to be done. I did not want a relationship with Bartee to distract my healing and serving Christ.

First, I took off my false eyelashes and my wig and I told him:

"I have Alopecia. It is a non-contagious autoimmune disease that means my body attacks my hair. My hair does not grow like it grows for other people and when it does grow in patches, it hurts and scars me. I am a bald woman"

Second, I told him:

"I have a mental illness. I have tried to commit suicide three times in my life. I maintain my mental health by serving Jesus, healthy living, through medication, counseling and family support. I have major depression and generalized anxiety disorder."

Bartee's response to both of my statements could have ONLY come from God, because he said exactly what I needed to hear. Bartee said:

"What do I do if you get sick?"

He also gave me a cute compliment on my bald head. He said that I look like a "China-Baby," but that's a story you will have to read in our other book (LOL!)

It feels good to laugh. It feels even better to have someone to laugh with! I have been blessed to cry, and now, I am being blessed to laugh. God has seen me through the fire of mental health hell, and He is soaking me up with His mighty garden hose! I am blessed not only because:

- God sent Bartee to find, date, and marry me in less than six months.

- God also blessed me to become a #1 Best-selling Author on Amazon.

- God blessed me to become a homeowner just months after Bartee and I married!

- God enlarged my territory as a business owner.

- God allowed me to serve as His anointed vessel, for His purpose, and to do His will!

- God anointed my voice like never before, and I become an audiobook publisher.

Now that Bartee has retired from 30-plus years as a Volusia County employee in the State of Florida, we plan to go on tour testifying on the goodness of the Lord; sharing music and books; bringing our workshops and conferences; and enjoying each other.

If you are in that dark place now, hold on to God's hand; it NEVER changes, His hand NEVER leaves you, it NEVER forgets about you. He is there for you if you ask Him. Now, it may take YOU a bit of time to feel His presence or hear His voice, but allow yourself all of the time that you need.

Don't give up.

Don't let someone else make you feel like you need to "get over it."

Don't get "tired."

Don't forget my story.

It didn't take me ten years from attempted suicide to a shower of blessings. It really only took me a couple of years to learn my "triggers" and avoid them; it only took me a few months to begin to feel whole again. I am still learning! I recently learned what the term "gaslighting" means, and now I avoid those people and situations where I could be a victim of it.

Give yourself time to heal and learn, and give yourself time to receive God's love. You never know how your experiences and your story could help save the life of another.

Last Week...I Wanted to Die

CONTACT THE AUTHOR:

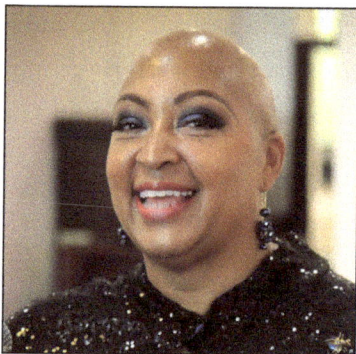

Angie BEE Productions

*Producing Christian entertainment enjoyed
by the entire family!*

*See our past projects at
www.YouTube.com/AngieBEEpresents
Facebook.com/AngieBEEproductions
Facebook.com/LastWeekIWantedToDie*

Visit us online today at
www.Facebook.com/DaQueenBeeEvangelistAngieBEE

www.DaQueenBee.com
Call us today at 407-914-6519 or send an email to
AngieBEEproductions@gmail.com

Angie BEE is available to speak to your group or at your event! More projects by Angie BEE are coming soon!

BEE Blessed!

www.ingramcontent.com/pod-product-compliance
Lightning Source LLC
Chambersburg PA
CBHW070031030426
42335CB00017B/2378